THE LYSINE-ARGININE SURVIVAL GUIDE

HOW TO PREVENT COLD SORES & HERPES OUTBREAKS NATURALLY

THE LYSINE-ARGININE BLOGGER

Copyright © 2024 The Lysine-Arginine Blogger

All rights reserved.

DISCLAIMER

All rights reserved. Without limiting the rights under the copyright reserved above, no part of this publication may be reproduced, stored in, or introduced into a retrieval system, or transmitted in any form or by any means (electronic, mechanical, photocopying, recording, or otherwise) without prior written permission. For permission requests, please contact: YouAreLoved@LysineArginineGuide.com

The publisher and the author are providing this book and its contents on an "as is" basis and make no representations or warranties of any kind with respect to this book or its contents. The publisher and the author disclaim all such representations and warranties, including but not limited to warranties of healthcare for a particular purpose. In addition, the publisher and the author assume no responsibility for errors, inaccuracies, omissions, or any other inconsistencies herein.

The content of this book is for informational purposes only and is not intended to diagnose, treat, cure, or prevent any condition or disease. By reading this book, you agree that you understand this book is not intended as a substitute for consultation with a licensed practitioner. Please consult with your own physician or healthcare specialist regarding any suggestions and recommendations made in this book. The use of this book implies your 100% acceptance of this disclaimer.

The publisher and the author make no guarantees concerning the level of success you may experience by following the advice and strategies contained in this book, and you accept the risk that results will differ for each individual.

YOU SHOULD ALWAYS CONSULT WITH A HEALTHCARE PROFESSIONAL BEFORE STARTING ANY DIET, EXERCISE PROGRAM, SUPPLEMENTATION OR MEDICATION PROGRAM.

CONTENTS

Introduction 1

Section 1: Herpes 101 and the Lysine-Arginine Connection 5

Section 2: Food List: Highest Lysine / Lowest Arginine 16

Section 3: Food List: Highest Arginine / Lowest Lysine 19

Section 4: Five Steps to an OB-Free Life 27

Section 5: Medications and Supplements 32

Section 6: Topical Treatment Options 39

Section 7: Wrap Up + Your Awesomeness Reminder 43

In Closing 46

INTRODUCTION

Dear Reader,

When I first started my Lysine Arginine Blog back in 2014, I had no idea I'd be writing a book like this. I had the herps for 2 years at that point, and had already learned about the "too much arginine = living hell" connection. I was painstakingly avoiding my favorite foods like peanut butter, Dave's Killer Bread (the 21 Whole Grains and Seeds one – sooo yummy), hummus, peanut butter, macadamia nuts, chocolate, peanut butter. Oh, and did I mention peanut butter? Because, peanut butter.

Anyway! The point is I knew to avoid foods with high levels of arginine. I had recently started weight training again and wanted to get back into making my protein smoothies. But when I started searching for a protein powder without arginine, it turned into a nightmare! I searched profusely, both in-person and online, only to come to the realization that (gasp!) it did not exist.

However, I learned that having arginine was okay, as long as you have lysine at the same time in an equal or larger amount. That's when things clicked for me and I started finding protein powders I could actually take without unleashing the fury within. It was a huge breakthrough and helped me SO MUCH. I couldn't wait to tell as many other people about it as possible. If I could save just one person from going through all of the pain, stress, and frustration that I went through, it would all be worth it.

So, I created this guide to answer a lot of the questions I've gotten over the years, and give you all of my best info in one straight shot, making your life easier, and hopefully preventing you from experiencing any more unnecessary pain and suffering.

I also wanted to help eliminate your frustration of trying to navigate the countless number of websites with contradicting information about which foods are herpes-friendly. It is absolute madness!

I'm sure these sites are well-intentioned, but for example, there's one site out there that says "eat more foods with B-vitamins" where they list berries, carrots, and mushrooms. Then in the next section, they say "avoid high arginine foods" where they list berries, carrots, and mushrooms! Are you freaking kidding me?! Who's writing this stuff?!

I wanted to give you all the exact opposite: A clear, straightforward guide with information that came from a reliable source. In order to do that, my Executive Assistant (ahem, ok, my incredibly supportive Mom!) and I researched every food listed in this book using the USDA's FoodData Central Database.

By the way, I also offer a companion guide to this book called ***The Lysine vs Arginine Food Ratio Charts*** that has 60+ pages of lysine and arginine ratios in common foods. (It is available on Amazon in both eBook and paperback formats.)

Before you dive in though, let's just touch base on what this book is and what this book isn't.

This book is NOT:

- Written by a medical doctor, a licensed nutritionist, or anyone with a really cool, fancy title.

- A textbook that contains the answer to every question ever asked or that ever will be asked about Herpes, Lysine, and Arginine.

- Formally written in perfect English, with formal grammar, and perfect punctuation.

This book IS:

- Written by a regular gal who has gone through the pain and suffering of the herps herself and wants to help prevent or eliminate it for as many others as she can.

- A complete starter guide for people with some form of the herpes virus, who are new to the connection between lysine, arginine, and outbreaks.

- Casually written in plain language with my quirky sense of humor sprinkled in for good measure.

A Quick Word on Terminology

Throughout this book, instead of using the word "herpes" I use "the herps." Why? Because it's funny and has no icky stigma attached to it. I feel like it helps to minimize the feeling of it being this big deal, which it really isn't (once you get control over it). Also, I'm sure you've seen it before, but just in case, I use "OB" which means "outbreak."

Finally, I am providing the information in this book from the perspective of my own experience, which is being diagnosed with the herpes simplex virus. (Technically HSV1, but you'll read more about that in Chapter 1!)

Although I can't speak from experience on these, I get emails from readers all over the world who are using this information to help with other viruses in the herpes family including Shingles and Epstein-Barr Virus (EBV). So, no matter what brought you to this book, I hope it helps you to find relief, peace, and healing.

Wishing You Vibrant Health,
The Lysine-Arginine Blogger

P.S. To save you from having to manually type in the URL of all of the website links mentioned in this book, please visit the page below for clickable links of each URL mentioned:

https://www.LysineArginineGuide.com/sources

SECTION 1

Herpes 101 and The Lysine-Arginine Connection

Okay, it's time to talk about our favorite topic: Herpes. Or as I like to call it, the herps! Oh alright, it might not be our favorite topic, but trust me, the more you learn, the more you will know, and that knowledge will help you experience more peace and a lot less pain and suffering.

So what is this thing called herpes anyway? I'm going to use my own words here, because most of the definitions I've come across online make it sound so icky, when it's really not. At the most basic level, herpes is a virus, period.

There are more than 100 known herpes viruses, of which only 8 of them routinely infect only humans. For our purposes here, we're only going to go over Herpes Simplex Virus 1 (HSV1) and Herpes Simplex Virus 2 (HSV2). (If you have a different one, I highly encourage you to do some research on it to help you understand how it works in the body!)

Once a person is infected with HSV1 or HSV2, the virus will generally create an initial freak out in the body (aka initial outbreak or "OB"). It will get into the nerve roots and head straight to one of two sensory nerve ganglion (which is a group of nerve cell bodies).

Type 1 usually goes and hangs out in the trigeminal ganglion, which is a collection of nerve cells located behind the cheekbone near the ear, and Type 2 usually goes to the sacral ganglion at the base of the spine. So that's the biggest difference, where it lives: near the ear or the base of the spine. Simple, right? Now, did you notice my key word usually? I said usually, because technically either one can hang out in either place. But, most commonly, Type 1 hangs out near the ear, and Type 2 hangs out near your tushy.

To be clear, there are some differences between them, but after doing a ton of research, most of the detailed, specific differences didn't really matter to me. I was just trying to figure out how to live with this thing called herpes, not be a molecular biologist.

It was so confusing when I first found out because my boyfriend at the time, who unknowingly passed it to me, tested positive for Type 2, but I tested positive for Type 1. I had my initial OB "down there," so I was like, "How is that possible?!"

I got equally confusing answers from my doctor - something about him maybe having Chicken Pox as a kid, antibodies not currently being active, blood tests not always being reliable, blah blah blah. She was basically like, "Let me say whatever I can to get this girl, who is having an emotional meltdown that I don't know how to deal with, out of my office asap."

So, because of the lack of answers from the doctor, I went down the "What type do I have??" rabbit hole for months, desperate to find out, and then came to this very simple conclusion: They both cause outbreaks, they both get triggered by the same things, and they both get treated with the same medications. That was enough for me, and is all I've needed to know to thrive with the herps, regardless of whether I have Type 1, Type 2, or both.

Important Stuff You Should Know

In rare cases, both HSV1 and HSV2 can potentially infect the eye, which leads to blindness if not treated. They can also infect the brain, causing encephalitis, which can cause major problems and would need to be treated asap. It is much more common for HSV1 to infect these areas, but HSV2 can do it as well. Again these occurrences are rare, but important for you to be aware of.

Another thing to be aware of is herpes and pregnancy. If a woman becomes pregnant after already having herpes, the doctors will be on the lookout for signs of an outbreak near delivery, and if that's the case, the baby may likely be delivered via C-section to prevent it from being passed on to the baby. If a woman is already pregnant and then gets herpes, there can be severe complications. In either case, it's important to have doctors involved at each step, to prevent passing it to the baby, and thereby preventing any lifelong complications that may occur.

H Prodrome: Common OB Warning Signs

If you've had the herps for years, you probably know exactly when it's about to throw a coming out party on your face or in your tighty whiteys. However, if you're a newbie, you might still be figuring it out. I'm mentioning it here because it's important for you to really get to know your body and how it signals you of when an OB is coming so you can:

1. Do what you need to prevent it asap.
2. Figure out what the heck might have caused it.

The more you are able to connect the dots between your OBs and your triggers, the more you will be able to reduce and prevent them altogether.

The term "prodrome" refers to symptoms that occur before an illness. For example, people that suffer from migraines may start to exhibit symptoms such as nausea and sensitivity to light before the actual migraine hits. Those symptoms would be considered migraine prodrome.

The herps has its own set of prodrome symptoms and thank goodness it does! They might be uncomfortable, but they are blessings in disguise. They give you a lovely heads up so you can take action and prevent any embarrassing situations as well as additional pain and suffering if you are able to nip it in the bud.

Here are the most common Herpes prodrome symptoms (a.k.a. OB warning signs):

- Tingling, itching, or burning sensations near the surface of the skin

- Painful nerve sensations in the lower back, buttocks, or thighs

- Body aches

- Fatigue

- Swollen lymph nodes

- Flu-like symptoms

- Headache

I haven't had an OB in quite a while, but I always knew when one was coming on. Mine would usually start with me feeling extremely fatigued, like I was coming down with a cold, especially when I woke up in the morning. It would be followed by a tingling sensation in my left tushy cheek (ok, ok "buttock" lol) that would become achy and painful, and travel down my leg. If I didn't take medicine, it would become so unbearable that I could hardly walk.

Note of Encouragement: Writing this section has reminded me of how far I have come. My life felt like a living hell at one point because of the herps and now I barely even think about it! So don't give up! There is nothing special about me. If I can learn and take action to be OB-free, so can you! If you read and follow everything in this guidebook, you will be well on your way to an OB-free future, and let me tell you, it is AWESOME.

Other Things That Can Trigger OBs

In addition to high arginine levels in food, there are other things that can trigger OBs, including certain supplements. Supplements are reviewed in more detail in Chapter 6, but here are some other things that can cause OBs that you should be aware of.

- Stress (For REAL peeps. Imho, stress is right up there with arginine. See the Special Note below.)
- Coming down with a cold/flu or being around someone that has one
- Not getting enough sleep / Physical Exhaustion
- Weakened Immune System
- Physical Trauma (a major injury, surgery, etc.)
- Sun exposure or tanning beds (UV Light)
- Laser Hair Removal
- Strong wind that can cause chapped lips (For those that get cold sores on/around the lips)
- Medications that suppress the immune system
- Friction from sexual activity or intercourse
- Hormonal fluctuations

SPECIAL NOTE: Nervous System Regulation

Regarding the connection between stress and OB's, if you are struggling with constant OB's or are dealing with any chronic illness, you might want to look into the concept of nervous system regulation.

I have been studying this topic and practically applying what I've been learning for a few years now, and the results I've experienced have been life-changing on so many levels.

It goes beyond things like meditation, relaxation, etc and helps the body heal by establishing regulation in the nervous system; where the root of the problem exists.

If you'd like to learn more, below are a few resources from Irene Lyon, MSC. She is a Nervous System Expert and Master Somatic Practitioner. I researched a number of teachers, and while there are many on this topic, I found her teachings to be the most thorough and complete.

She combines her own experiences working with clients with the findings of a number of top teachers and pioneers in the field to create her educational materials. She is also highly skilled at breaking down complex concepts and translating them into language that's easy to understand.

Reminder: Clickable links of all URLS can be found on this page of the blog: https://www.LysineArginineGuide.com/sources

How Stored Trauma Creates Somatic Symptoms (aka Chronic Illness)
URL: https://bit.ly/irene-trauma-1

The Connection Between Traumatic Stress and Chronic Illness
URL: https://bit.ly/irene-trauma-2

The 2nd video is less polished than what she's publishing now, but it's the video that caused a huge AHA moment for me, so I have to include it. It enabled me to put the all the pieces of my entire health journey together (going back to childhood) and set me on the wonderful path of (complete) healing I'm on now.

Testimonial: This is a testimonial from one of her students who stopped having herpes outbreaks as a result of establishing more regulation in her nervous system.

URL: https://bit.ly/irene-student-1

Be sure to click the arrow on the right side of the image to read each slide.

Is There a Cure for the Herps?

Depending on who you ask, you will get very different answers to this question. If you ask most people in the medical community, you will most likely hear, "No. You can suppress it with medication, but it is incurable."

If you ask the loyal online followers of Dr. Boogidybooboo (ok I made that one up, but insert your favorite fake doctor's name here), you will hear, "yes! i am so grateful to God!!!! i testify Dr.Boogidybooboo cure my herpes virus within 5 days!!!! call him whatsapp or email him and he cure you too!!!"

However, if you ask someone like me, you will hear "Not yet, but it's on the way." Oh yes, mark my words. I 100% believe there will be a cure for the herps someday. There is so much progress being made and advances occurring in medical research and technology that I believe a cure is inevitable. It's not a question of if, it's a question of when.

Here are just a couple of resources to check out to learn more:

DRACO by MIT graduate Dr. Todd Rider:
- **Video explaining DRACO**: https://bit.ly/draco-video
- **The Rider Institute: All about DRACO Broad-Spectrum Antiviral Therapeutics:** https://riderinstitute.org/discovery

CRISPR / Genetic Engineering:
- Video about CRISPR + genetic engineering: https://bit.ly/4dRofL5

That link will take you straight to the part about its potential for curing diseases and viruses.

Heads Up: "Herpes Cure" Scam Alert!

When I was first diagnosed and in a state of utter despair, I spent $67 on a stupid e-book that claimed it had the cure for the herps. The video I watched told me that the evil pharmaceutical companies were hiding the cure from me, and that over 27,000 people had already healed themselves using the information in the book.

But it was crrrrrap! Crap I tell you! It was a total scam designed to get money from sad, scared people in a state of desperation, which is exactly where I was, and is exactly why they got me. I have since seen multiple similar e-books, and they have all had the same *extremely convincing* marketing scheme behind them.

So keep your spidey senses on high alert and don't fall for those e-book cure scams!

The Lysine-Arginine Connection

Ok, hopefully that gave you a basic idea of what the herps is. Now, what the heck are lysine and arginine and how are they connected to the herps?

In short, lysine (a.k.a. L-Lysine – pronounced LIE-SEEN) and arginine (a.k.a. L-Arginine – pronounced AR-JEN-EEN)) are 2 of 20 amino acids that are the building blocks that make up your body's proteins. So, your body needs both of them.

Lysine is an essential amino acid, meaning that your body cannot make it on its own, so you need to get it through the food you eat.

Arginine is a conditional amino acid, meaning that the body makes it on its own, and would only need to be intentionally consumed if the body wasn't making it sufficiently (e.g. in certain cases of illness or stress).

However, consuming too much arginine causes the herps to replicate, which greatly increases the chance of an OB. So technically, arginine doesn't cause the OB itself. What it does is feed the herps, giving it exactly what it needs to multiply like crazy and throw an unwanted party in your body. On the other hand, lysine blocks the activity of arginine, which helps to prevent the herps from replicating.

There are a number of scientific articles written on the antagonistic relationship between lysine and arginine, but honestly they are highly technical and hard for the average person to understand.

If you are a not scientist, but you think like one, do some internet searching, you'll find them! However, for most people who want to learn more, I would recommend reading this article:

Why We Need a High Lysine Diet by Joan Tendler, M.Arch
URL: httpss://bit.ly/3V42QGZ

It's a long read and ventures slightly into the realm of more complex concepts, but is the easiest article to read on the topic that I've found so far.

Ok, for now, let's work with the basic concept of what we know: Consuming too much arginine and not enough lysine can trigger an OB. With that knowledge, we have something to work with. Where it can get confusing is when you try to start finding out how much lysine and arginine are in certain foods so you know what to eat and what to avoid. In the next few chapters, we'll dive into exactly that.

SECTION 2

Food List: Highest Lysine / Lowest Arginine

All of the information in this section and the next were taken from *The Lysine vs Arginine Food Ratio Charts* I mentioned earlier. However, in the charts on the following pages, some things have been abbreviated for the sake of easy reading and formatting. For example, "Rice, brown, long- grain, cooked" was shortened to "Brown Rice" and measurement details like "whole" and "chopped" have been omitted.

Below is a list of foods that have some of the best (highest lysine to arginine) ratios. They all have at least twice the amount of lysine as they do arginine. Don't worry, you can eat a lot more food than this! These are just some of the most common foods with the best ratios, shown with the highest lysine to arginine ratio at the top.

Description	Weight (In grams)	Measure	Lysine(mg) Per Measure	Arginine(mg) Per Measure	Ratio Lysine to Arginine
Carambola (Starfruit)	132	1.0 cup	102	28	3.6 to 1
Yogurt, Greek, plain, lowfat	200	7 oz	942	316	3 to 1
Yogurt, plain, low fat	170	6 oz	801	269	3 to 1
Milk, 2%	244	1.0 cup	673	229	2.9 to 1
American Cheese	28.35	1.0 oz	430	147	2.9 to 1
Swiss Cheese	132	1.0 cup	3412	1224	2.8 to 1
Gouda Cheese	28.35	1.0 oz	752	273	2.8 to 1
Provolone Cheese	132	1.0 cup	3493	1349	2.6 to 1
Feta Cheese	150	1.0 cup	1829	705	2.6 to 1
Papayas	145	1.0 cup	36	14	2.6 to 1
Cauliflower	107	1.0 cup	232	92	2.5 to 1
Muenster Cheese	132	1.0 cup	2823	1163	2.4 to 1
Mozzarella Cheese	28.35	1.0 oz	699	295	2.4 to 1
Apricot	155	1.0 cup	150	70	2.1 to 1
Mango	165	1.0 cup	109	51	2.1 to 1
Apples	125	1.0 cup	15	7	2.1 to 1
Brown Mushrooms (Italian/Crimini)	87	1.0 cup	219	107	2 to 1
Portabella Mushrooms	86	1.0 cup	217	106	2 to 1

Note: To clarify any confusion about ratios, where it says "Lysine to Arginine," a 3 to 1 ratio means it has 3 times the amount of lysine than arginine.

A Note on Cheese and Yogurt

Every cheese listed in the USDA Food Composition Database has more lysine than arginine. I only listed the most common varieties with the highest lysine to arginine ratios.

Also, some fruit varieties of yogurt may contain gelatin, which is high in arginine. The amount of lysine may offset it, but if you're eating yogurt specifically for the lysine ratio, then it can defeat the purpose.

SECTION 3

Food List: Highest Arginine / Lowest Lysine

The chart on the following pages contains a list of foods that have a very high arginine to lysine ratio. They all have at LEAST twice the amount of arginine as they do lysine, so avoid them entirely or proceed with caution. The chart is sorted by ratio, with the highest arginine and lowest lysine ratio at the top.

IMPORTANT NOTE

This is the ONLY chart in the book that is sorted with the highest arginine foods at the top, and the far right "Ratio" column displaying Arginine to Lysine. I did this so it was easier for you to see exactly how much more arginine the food has vs lysine.

All other charts are sorted with the highest lysine to arginine ratio at the top, with the far right "Ratio" column displaying Lysine to Arginine.

Description	Weight (In Grams)	Measure	Lysine(mg) Per Measure	Arginine(mg) Per Measure	Ratio Arginine to Lysine
Macadamia Nuts	134	1.0 cup	24	1879	78.3 to 1
Hazelnuts	115	1.0 cup	483	2543	5.3 to 1
Orange Juice	248	1.0 cup	22	117	5.3 to 1
Walnuts (Black)	125	1.0 cup	891	4522	5.1 to 1
Raisins	165	1.0 cup	139	681	4.9 to 1
Tangerine Juice	247	1.0 cup	17	84	4.9 to 1
Grapes, red or green	151	1.0 cup	41	196	4.8 to 1
Grape Juice	253	1.0 cup	25	119	4.8 to 1
Sesame Seeds	144	1.0 cup	819	3787	4.6 to 1
Pine Nuts	135	1.0 cup	729	3258	4.5 to 1
Brazil Nuts	133	1.0 cup	652	2846	4.4 to 1
Grapefruit	230	1.0 cup	37	161	4.4 to 1
Pumpkin Seeds	129	1.0 cup	1594	6905	4.3 to 1
Almonds	143	1.0 cup	812	3525	4.3 to 1
Pecans	109	1.0 cup	313	1283	4.1 to 1
Peanut Butter	32	2.0 tbsp	218	886	4.1 to 1
Almond Butter	16	1.0 tbsp	98	381	3.9 to 1
Coconut Milk	240	1.0 cup	242	902	3.7 to 1

Avoid or use caution with these!

A Few Quick Touchpoints

Chocolate

Although there were numerous listings for chocolate in the USDA Food Composition Database, I was not able to find one that had the amino acid profile listed. However, chocolate is well-known within the herps community to cause OBs. It also contains caffeine, which can trigger OBs for some of us, so be super careful with it.

Nut Milks, Pesto, and Tahini

I didn't list all of the nut milks here, but don't forget about them. So things like almond milk and cashew milk are going to have more arginine than lysine as well. Also, don't forget that pesto is made with pine nuts and tahini is made with sesame seeds. Yes, both of those have snuck by me and hello holy ravenous herpalicious disco party in my pants.

Coconut Water

I have come across lots of sites that say coconut water is fine to drink if you have the herps. One site even groups it with coconut oil and says, "Coconut water and coconut oil have no proteins or amino acids and will not affect the herpes virus." However, my research shows differently. While the USDA Food Composition Database does not have amino acid profiles available for coconut oil, it does have a listing for coconut water, and it is shown to have approximately 3 times the amount of arginine than lysine.

So, I would recommend avoiding it until one of those well-meaning people can verify where they are getting their information from. Also, there are a few listings for coconut flour in the USDA Food Composition database, but they do not provide the amino acid profiles. However, I think it's safe to assume that since coconut meat and milk are both high in arginine and low in lysine, coconut flour is as well.

Oils

In addition to searching the USDA Food Composition Database, I have also read numerous articles from multiple sources, and everything I read indicated that oils do not contain the amino acids lysine or arginine, including coconut oil, so they will not trigger an OB.

Other Foods that Can Cause OBs

Even though these foods might not contain arginine, they may trigger OBs for other reasons.

- Caffeine
- Spicy Foods
- Artificial Sweeteners
- Watermelon, melon, cantaloupe, cucumber

I personally stopped consuming artificial sweeteners a long time ago, so I can't personally attest to whether or not it causes OBs, but I can definitely attest to both caffeine and spicy foods causing them.

I tend to be super sensitive to caffeine anyway, like one cup of black tea would give me the shakes, have me talking like Six from Blossom, and then the next day, an OB would sparkle its way to the surface of my hoo ha like a dancing unicorn.

Same thing with spicy foods. I realized that one after living in California and making the connection between Taco Tuesday and OB Wednesday. It was kind of like getting the toy from a Happy Meal, except I got it the next day, and instead of a toy it was a mini mariachi band called "Los Herpecitos en Tus Chonecitos" singing their greatest hits in my underpants. Remember though, every body is different, so just because they caused OBs for me, doesn't necessarily mean they will cause OBs for you.

Another thing I wanted to mention is that I came across a few sites that said watermelon, melon, cantaloupe, and cucumber may contribute to causing OBs, not necessarily because of the actual arginine content, but because they contain something called citrulline, which may contribute to the body's own production of arginine.

The theory comes from a study done by the Journal of Nutrition, which was done on mice. I personally haven't noticed any OBs from eating watermelon, melon, cantaloupe, or cucumber, but I also don't eat a large amount of them or even eat them regularly.

I wanted to mention it here though, because if you are consuming any of them frequently or in large amounts, and are having OBs, then it might be something to experiment with. Try eliminating them or reducing the amount you're eating for a while, and see if it makes a difference.

Some Things to Keep in Mind:
Ratio, Quantity, and Combination

Ratio

When analyzing lysine/arginine food ratios, remember that it's possible for something to be both high in lysine and high in arginine. You always want to look at the *ratio* of lysine to arginine, with more lysine than arginine being the goal in order to prevent OBs.

For example, one cup of chickpeas (a.k.a. garbanzo beans) has 973mg of lysine, which is high compared to something like cherry tomatoes, which only has 40mg of lysine per cup.

However, one cup of chickpeas also has 1369mg of arginine, compared to cherry tomatoes, which only have 31mg of arginine per cup.

So in a case like this, even though chickpeas technically have more lysine than cherry tomatoes, I consider them to be a high-arginine food, and tomatoes a high-lysine food because of the ratios.

So, for our purposes, more lysine than arginine = "high lysine food" and more arginine than lysine = "high arginine food."

Ratio Example:

Food	Lysine (mg) per cup	Arginine (mg) per cup
Chickpeas	973	1369
Cherry Tomatoes	40	31

Quantity

When deciding whether to eat a certain food depending on its lysine and arginine content, always consider the quantity you're going to be consuming before deciding whether or not to eat it.

For example, if you look at the table below, you will see that garlic has quite a bit more arginine than lysine. But have you ever eaten a CUP of garlic in one sitting with no other food? Probably not. Chances are you combined it with other foods, which is what we touch on next.

Quantity Example:

Food	Weight (In Grams)	Measure	Lysine (mg) Per Measure	Arginine (mg) Per Measure	Ratio Lysine to Arginine
Garlic	136	1.0 cup	371	862	0.4 to 1

Combination

Also, just because a food has more arginine than lysine, that doesn't mean you should avoid it completely. I personally would recommend staying away from the foods with the highest arginine to lysine ratio (like nuts) because it's harder to offset them. However, foods that have somewhat more arginine than are easier to offset with other foods that have more lysine than arginine.

For example, a meal could look like this:

Food	Weight (In grams)	Measure	Lysine (mg) Per Measure	Arginine (mg) Per Measure
Chicken Breast	85	3.0 oz	2496	1755
Grilled Onions	105	½ Cup	69	192
Broccoli	91	1.0 cup chopped	123	174
Sweet Potato	200	1.0 cup	168	140
TOTALS:			2856	2261

So, you can see from the above example that even though onions and broccoli have more arginine than lysine, they are easily offset by the additional lysine in the chicken and in the sweet potato.

There are some foods that don't have a huge amount more arginine than lysine, but are commonly eaten alone and can still cause OBs if they are. I have personally made the mistake of eating them alone and not combining them with other higher lysine foods to offset the arginine. The result? OB city all up in my skivvies. Lesson learned! Here are some of them:

- Lentils
- Oats and Oatmeal
- Quinoa
- Hummus (made from chickpeas)

Pasta and wheat products, including food made with white flour, all have more arginine than lysine, so be careful eating them alone. Also, I know it's hard, but eliminating refined, processed foods from your diet yet (like white bread, cookies, sugar cereals, etc.) is really an excellent thing to do for your immune system and overall health. Your body will only be as healthy and vibrant as the foods you put in it, and will reward you for it with a better feeling body, and less OBs!

SECTION 4

Five Steps to an OB-Free Life

As you start to eat more consciously to prevent OBs, I want to encourage you to approach it from a macro-view perspective. Try to think about your body and your health from a holistic point of view.

Study this guidebook and gain a good solid understanding of what to eat and what to avoid. Then, rather than obsessing about the specific lysine/arginine ratios of every single food, just focus on avoiding high-arginine, low lysine foods, eating fresh, whole foods (preferably organic), eat less processed foods, and avoid triggers.

You want your focus to be on experiencing vibrant, overall health, not just eating to prevent outbreaks. You want your immune system and your whole body to be strong and healthy. The stronger and healthier your immune system and body is as a whole, the less OBs you will experience. My absolute best advice to you, to free yourself from OBs, is to follow these basic 5 steps.

Five Steps to an OB-Free Life:

1. Avoid foods and supplements that are high in arginine and low in lysine.

2. Look for and eliminate any other possible triggers (See Chapter 5).

3. Regularly implement fun or stress-relieving activities to keep your stress levels low.

4. Take a "food as medicine" approach to eating. Replace processed foods with fresh, healthy, whole foods, and go organic as much as you possibly can.

5. Take medication and/or supplements and use topical treatments as needed.

When you're trying to eliminate OBs from your life, I recommend following those 5 steps in order. Start by eliminating the triggers, strengthen your body and immune system by eating good, healthy food and keeping your stress levels manageable, and take medicine and/or supplements if and when you need them.

I recommend following that order because if you just go straight to medicine or supplements and your OBs are being caused by eating a certain food, then you are going to be wasting your money and putting extra stuff in your body that's not necessary.

Also, please don't forget about nervous system regulation. It goes beyond the simplicity of what I mention in Step 3 regarding stress, and can help you to experience lasting healing because it works at a foundational, root-cause level.

So What CAN You Eat?

My best recommendation is for you to eat as much fresh, whole foods (preferably organic) as you can. This is because processed and packaged foods do not contain the vital life force nutrients that our bodies need to function at the optimal level they were designed to.

Whole food options include:

- Vegetables (Especially ones that contain I3C – See below)
- Fruits
- Eggs
- Dairy

- Meat
- Whole Grains (Minimally processed and only if your body can tolerate them and you combine them intelligently.)

Regardless of whether you eat meat or not, if you stick to eating whole foods and avoid processed foods and known OB-Trigger foods, you are setting yourself up for success: a healthy body that feels good and is much less likely to have OBs.

However, if you are not eating a lot of whole foods right now, don't think you have to swing to the total opposite end of the spectrum and eat only100% fresh, organic, whole food starting tomorrow morning. You can of course, but just know it's okay to take your time and slowly implement one or two foods a week.

Just start adding them to your routine so you can get used to them. Then, slowly add a little more. Over time, you will find your body craving them, and before you know it, your eating habits will be completely transformed.

A Simple Habit to Help You Eat Healthier Right Away

A few years ago, I came across a fantastic book called Simple Green Smoothies by Jen Hansard and Jadah Sellner. I truly cannot say enough about this book. It LIVES on my kitchen counter.

Their encouraging and highly realistic approach to establishing a healthy lifestyle really inspired me. It was basically this: drink a green smoothie every day. Super simple, right?? I researched tons of books before finding that one, and let me tell you, it is a true GEM.

The book gives awesome advice about making smoothies (including the best blender options, the best order to put the ingredients in the blender, serving sizes, mix and match fruit/veggie charts, etc!!), but it also has tons of recipes with beautiful pictures, plus a 10-Day Kickstart to get you into the smoothie- making habit.

These ladies are the queens of smoothie making and I highly recommend the book as a way to start transitioning into a more whole foods based lifestyle. (You can add your favorite high-lysine protein powder to your smoothies!)

Cruciferous Veggies + Indole-3-Carbinol (I3C)

There are a growing number of studies, including one done by Northeastern Ohio Universities College of Medicine, indicating eating broccoli, can help to inhibit the herps from replicating due to a compound called Indole-3-Carbinol (I3C).

The study states, "We have discovered that this relatively nontoxic compound found in certain foods inhibits HSV replication by at least 99.9% in vitro in tissue culture." I3C can also be found in other cruciferous vegetables, such as brussels sprouts, cauliflower, cabbage, kale, mustard greens, watercress, kohlrabi, and bok choi.

Of course, I encourage you to eat as much of those as you can (organic if possible), but I3C is also available in supplement form if you would like to try it.

SECTION 5

Medications and Supplements

Medications

I'm not going to talk too much about medications here because there's lots of info online, but I'll give you a quick review and tell you a little bit about my personal experience. First of all, the most popular prescription medications used to treat and suppress the herps are shown in the chart below.

Generic Name	Brand Name
Acyclovir	Zovirax
Valacyclovir	Valtrex
Famciclovir	Famvir
Penciclovir (Cream)	Denavir

*Acyclovir / Zovirax is also available as a cream and ointment.

For me personally, changing my diet by eliminating high arginine, low lysine foods, eating more healthy, whole foods, and effectively managing my stress level eliminated 99% of my OBs. I would still get the occasional OB with my monthly cycle though, so I took the advice of my best friend who also has the herps!). She encouraged me to get the medication and keep it on hand for those fun times. My doctor prescribed Valacyclovir for me and it worked like a charm whenever I needed it.

However, if you're on high blood pressure medication, your doctor may prescribe the cream or ointment instead of the oral medication to prevent any interactions. This is what another one of my friends is doing and she says the cream works significantly better and faster than any of the over-the-counter topical treatments she was previously using, including the ones I mention coming up in Chapter 6.

If you go the prescription medication route, you might want to skip the over-the-counter treatments and go straight for the prescription cream. This could also be a great option for someone who isn't on any medication that might cause interactions, but who simply would rather apply a cream or ointment than take a pill.

Just remember the OB has to be in a spot that's conducive to a topical treatment. You may have to cover it with a non-stickbandage pad so it doesn't get absorbed through your clothes and show on the outside. ("No, I didn't sit in anything. That's just my herpes cream!" LOL. Yeah, let's skip that convo, shall we?)

Supplements

When it comes to the herps, there's a snake oil seller at every corner, so don't believe everything you read. Like I mentioned before, I know there is a cure coming for the herps, I am certain of that, but I do not believe it exists yet. However, in addition to or as an alternative to medication, there are supplements that can help keep it at bay and discourage the occurrence of OBs.

In my honest opinion though, I would not rely solely on supplements to help you if you are having recurring OBs. Meaning, if you are eating a diet with higher levels of arginine than lysine, plus processed foods, sugar, and all the other stuff being sold in grocery stores today and are having recurring OBs, I would make changing your diet priority numero uno. I'm not saying *not* to take supplements; I'm saying it wouldn't make sense to *just* take supplements and not change your diet, since the diet could be the culprit of the recurring OBs.

It's so easy to get caught up in the hamster wheel of supplement land, going from one supplement to another, hoping the next one will do the trick, while you stuff your mouth with what equates to candy for arginine. That being said, in this section we'll touch on some supplement options and some things to look out for.

Supplements That Can Help

Lysine

This one gets its own section because it is the most popular, and potentially the most effective supplement in dealing with the herps. In my own personal experience, and feedback from my readers, lysine is best at *preventing* OBs versus treating them. However, if you take it *as soon as* you feel like you might be getting one, it can either prevent it from happening altogether or at least reduce the severity and length of the OB. Most who supplement with lysine do A, B, or C as follows:

A) Take it on a daily basis as a preventative.

B) Only take it as soon as they feel an OB coming on.

C) Take it on a daily basis, then increase the dosage if they feel an OB coming on.

If you want to try taking lysine, you'll have to test to see what works for you. However, here are common dosages to give you an idea of where to start:

Preventative: 500-1000mg taken once per day everyday.

OB Coming: 1000mg taken three times per day for the duration of the OB.

Although it is very common for people to take lysine every day, long-term effects of daily lysine supplementation have not been determined yet. There are also many recommendations that say you should not take lysine if you have problems with your kidneys or liver, if you have hyperlysinemia/hyperlysinuria, and if you are pregnant or lactating. **As always, talk to your doctor to be safe.**

Forms of Lysine

As an internal supplement, (versus a topical application – See "Section 7: Topical Treatment Options"), lysine comes in powder, chewables, liquid extract, or pill form (tablets, caplets, capsules).

When I first started making smoothies again after my lysine/arginine discovery, I tried adding lysine powder to my smoothies, and holy bubbles Batman, trouble in Belly Town. Big trouble. The kind that can cause major problems if you need to actually function in society by leaving your house and being around other people (and not have your tushy glued to the porcelain throne all day). However, I tried Super Lysine + by Quantum Health (recommended by my awesome readers!) and it caused no negative effects for me.

Again, every body is different, so the powder might be okay for you, but based on my experience and the feedback from my readers, Super Lysine + seems like a better option. What makes it different from other lysine supplements is that in addition to lysine, it also contains Vitamin C, Echinacea, Licorice, and Propolis which help support the immune system.

Some other popular supplements to help prevent OBs:

- Astragalus
- B-Complex*
- Bioflavonoids
- Calendula
- Echinacea
- Indole-3-Carbinol (I3C)
- Licorice Root
- Oil of Oregano
- Olive Leaf Extract
- Propolis
- Red Marine Algae
- Turmeric Extract
- Vitamin C
- Zinc

B-Complex Caution: I tried taking B-Complex and it caused me to have heart flutters and palpitations, so I stopped it immediately. Again, with this or any other supplement, it's always helpful to be under the care of a doctor (western medicine, functional medicine, Chinese Medicine, Naturopaths, etc.) so you can get advice on what to take and feedback whenever you have a weird reaction.

Protein Powders

This book would not be complete without me mentioning protein powders! If you've read my blog, then you know that's where this whole journey started for me. I wanted to start lifting weights again, so I started making protein smoothies... and then started having non-stop OBs because my protein powder had an enormous amount of arginine in it and not a lot of lysine.

Once I figured that part out, and finally found a protein powder that had more lysine than arginine (and met my other requirements), I couldn't WAIT to tell the world about it and the blog was born. A lot of protein powders contain more arginine than lysine, so make sure to read the label, and if it doesn't list amino acids, don't buy it! (In case you're curious, my current favorite is Levels Protein Powder.)

Supplements to Avoid

Here are some other type of supplements that might contain arginine, even if it's not listed on the label. The following list doesn't indicate it definitely has arginine; it means that it *might*. So be sure to check and read all of the ingredients if you're interested in taking one of these supplements.

- Those labeled "Muscle-Building"
- Some "Pre-Workout" and "Post-Workout" formulas

- Some "Erectile Dysfunction" supplements
- Some "Fertility" supplements

The supplements below either are highly likely to have large amounts of arginine themselves or are known to elevate arginine levels in the body and cause OBs for some, so avoid them completely or be super careful.

- Citrulline
- Collagen
- Nitric Oxide / NO2
- Some Creatine Supplements

Also, watch out for capsules in general (versus tablets and caplets) because they may contain gelatin, and therefore, arginine. So make sure you read all ingredients. Those that say "Vegetarian Capsules," "Vegetable Capsules" or "Vegetable Cellulose" do not contain gelatin. In theory, taking a lysine supplement in a gelatin capsule should be fine because of the lysine to arginine ratio, but when there are other options, why add to your arginine load if you don't have to?

Special Mention: Elderberry

Elderberry is something I've seen a lot of sites recommend as a way to prevent OBs because it is considered to be a powerful anti-viral. However, Elderberry made my herps throw a disco party, invite all its friends, and do a group sing-along to "Ain't No Stopping Us Now." (Thanks to people who write "helpful" articles for people with herpes but who have no clue about arginine!!)

It has almost twice the amount of arginine than lysine, and I had no idea. It took me about 3 or 4 crazy OBs to finally make the connection and realize that's what was triggering them. Hopefully this will prevent you from having the same experience!

SECTION 6

Topical Treatment Options

For the first couple of years after getting diagnosed, I tried quite a few topical treatments and none of them really knocked my socks off. Keep in mind though that my OBs always happened below the belt, either on my tush, in the same exact spot, or on my hoo-ha, also usually in the same exact spot.

Both areas are difficult to put anything on because: 1) You have to actually cover those areas with those things called clothes so you don't freak out the entire world and 2) The clothes you put on those areas do nothing but rub-a-dub-dub all day, removing and absorbing whatever you put on and creating that lovely almost unbearable sense of friction that just makes the whole freaking thing worse.

The only exception I would make here is Aloe Vera because it does tend to dry faster than most, but then, at least for me, it just made it more itchy (which is the last thing you need!).

My advice would be for you to try the ones you feel called to and see what works. If your OBs are also below the belt, unless you can spend the entire day with the OB out in the open with nothing covering it, I would stay away from Manuka Honey.

Tea Tree Oil smells VERY strong, so keep that in mind if you're going to be around other people. I never tried Propolis (a waxy substance made by honeybees), but it has been scientifically studied and shown to heal the OBs faster.

Now, I want to mention one that my Mom swears by. She's been using it for years and says it cuts her healing time in half. If you want to try it, it's made by the same company I mentioned before, though this one is a topical ointment: Quantum Health Lip Clear Lysine+. If you try it, let me know if it works for you too!

Natural Topical Treatments Options

- Aloe Vera
- Coconut Oil / Monolaurin
- Epsom Salt (Soaking in a bath with it)
- Lemon Balm (Melissa officinalis)
- Lysine
- Manuka Honey
- Neem Oil
- Propolis
- Tea Tree Oil
- Visarpa Clay
- Vitamin C
- Zinc

Keep in mind these are not "FDA Approved," they are considered "Nutritional Supplements."

Most Popular Over-the-Counter Topical Medication Options

- Abreva
- Releev
- Zilactin

Topical Treatment Options That I Do NOT Recommend

I do not recommend the treatments below either because of potential danger (I've read horror stories) or they are simply ineffective.

- Baking Soda
- BHT
- DMSO
- Hydrogen Peroxide
- ChoRaphoR™ (Contains copper sulfate, which the FDA deems as toxic.)

Topical Treatment for Post-OB Scarring

Although not a topical treatment for the herps itself, Mederma is a topical gel that has been super effective for me at reducing the skin discoloration/scarring that can occur after an OB.

As I mentioned before, I used to break out on my left tushy cheek in the same exact place and it would always leave a mark while the skin was healing and for months after. Not sexy!

When I started applying Mederma twice a day right after the OB healed (meaning no more open skin), the discoloration went away a LOT faster – weeks instead of months.

SECTION 7

Wrap Up + Your Awesomeness Reminder

You made it!

I truly hope this book has provided you with valuable information, given you a sense of relief, and even empowerment over this little thing called the herps. I know it can feel like a huge problem at first, but once you educate yourself and know what you need to do, you'll find it's really not a big deal at all. Imho, once you get your OBs under control, the only reason it can still seem like a big deal is because of the ridiculous stigma that has been associated with it.

According to Stanford University, the herps has been around since as early as ancient Greek times. However, the stigma has only been around for a few decades, most likely due to an antiviral drug marketing campaign that ran in the 1970s and 1980s. Movies and TV shows have continued to fuel the stigma though, which I find so ironic. Think about how many people working on those movies and TV shows have the herps themselves!

To put it into perspective for you, the World Health Organization estimates that globally, 3.7 BILLION people under 50 have Type 1 of the herps, and an estimated 417 MILLION people between the ages of 15 and 49 have Type 2 of the herps. That's 2 out of 3 people for Type 1 and 1 out of 5 or 6 people for Type 2. AND it's estimated that between 80-90% of people who have the herps don't even know they have it!

So, don't fret, you are far from being alone. All kinds of people from all walks of life have the herps and having it doesn't make you bad, dirty, or broken. What used to help me when I first found out was, wherever I went, I would count the people around me according to the statistics and be like, "Yep! Herps, herps, herps, herps . . ." LOL. It helped me to realize how incredibly common it was, and that people all around me really did have the herps, just like me. We're just not wearing t-shirts that announce it.

If you're still in the early stages of finding out about the herps, make sure you do whatever you need to process any emotions about it and come to a healthy acceptance. A phenomenal resource that I highly recommend is a The (H) Opportunity (www.herpesopportunity.com). It was created by Adrial Dale and it provides lots of free resources, including a support forum.

You can also talk with people you trust, go to a Herpes Support Group (www.hwerks.com/local-herpes-groups), journal about it, kick the crap out of a punching bag, whatever you have to do to accept it and come to peace about it. After a while, you'll see that it's really no biggie.

So here are my final words for you my friend: Everything is going to be okay. You are okay. You are a beautiful human being. You are not broken. You are not dirty. You are not a bad person. Having the herps is a teeny, tiny dot in the big picture of who you are and all that you will experience and accomplish in your life. The force of life that is innately within you and that seeks to express through you every day is more powerful than any adversity you could ever face.

Wishing You Vibrant Health,
The Lysine-Arginine Blogger

IN CLOSING

Dear Reader,

I'm committed to making this book as helpful as possible for you. If you have an idea on how it can be improved, please email me at: YouAreLoved@LysineArginineGuide.com

One more thing! Reviews are very helpful for independent authors. I would be so grateful if you left a review.

Thank you and wishing you vibrant health!

The Lysine-Arginine Blogger

P.S. Don't forget! Clickable links of all URLs mentioned in this book as well as a list of source articles can be found at: https://www.LysineArginineGuide.com/sources

Sources:

https://fdc.nal.usda.gov/

http://lpi.oregonstate.edu/mic/dietary-factors/phytochemicals/indole-3-carbinol

http://projectaccept.org/herpes-stigma-the-origin

http://scienceline.org/2013/10/herpes

http://www.scarleteen.com/article/bodies/this_is_about_genital_herpes

http://accurateclinic.com/wp-content/uploads/2016/02/Lemon-balm-University-of-Maryland-Medical-Center.pdf

https://altmedrev.com/wp-content/uploads/2019/02/v12-2-169.pdf

https://www.who.int/news/item/01-05-2020-billions-worldwide-living-with-herpes

https://www.who.int/news-room/fact-sheets/detail/herpes-simplex-virus

https://academic.oup.com/jn/article/147/4/596/4584706

https://medlineplus.gov/druginfo/natural/875.html

https://medlineplus.gov/ency/article/002222.htm

https://virus.stanford.edu/herpes/History.html

https://www.aao.org/eye-health/diseases/herpes-keratitis

https://www.cdc.gov/std/herpes/stdfact-herpes-detailed.htm

https://www.drugs.com/npp/lysine.html

https://www.herpes-coldsores.com/diet_and_nutrition_with_herpes.htm

https://www.hopkinsmedicine.org/healthlibrary/conditions/nervous_system_disorders/herpes_meningoencephalitis_134,27

https://www.ncbi.nlm.nih.gov/pmc/articles/PMC3209744/

https://www.ncbi.nlm.nih.gov/pubmed/10782483

https://www.ncbi.nlm.nih.gov/pubmed/12396675

https://www.ncbi.nlm.nih.gov/pubmed/23885073

Printed in Great Britain
by Amazon